Dear Juliet,

You are such a special little girl, you are loved. You so mommy & daddy wanted you for a very long time. A lot of people prayed for you, and are so happy you are finally here. I hope this love story reminds you of all the love around you. Welcome to the world sweet, strong girl. Welco. to endless, unconditional love, and the BEST mommy, daddy a big brother you could dream of. Ho Baby

With love,
Auntie V,
& Uncle Jonathan

you were made for me

BY **SHERI STURNIOLO**

ILLUSTRATED BY

HANNAH PAK + SHAY LARBY

"Where once lay the heart of a couple,
now beats the heart of a family.
Forever and ever in our hearts you'll be."

Dedicated to all of the
wonderful fertility specialists that help
put the "pieces together"

YouWereMadeForMe.com

YOU WERE MADE FOR ME

BY **SHERI STURNIOLO**

ILLUSTRATED BY

HANNAH PAK +

SHAY LARBY

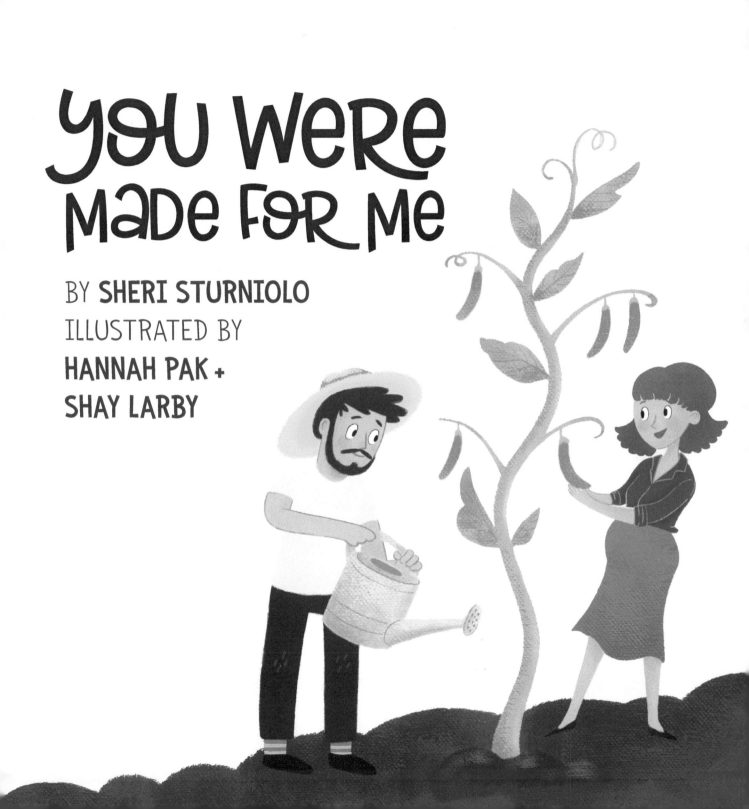

I'll tell you a story, amazing and true,
Of how you became the most wonderful you!

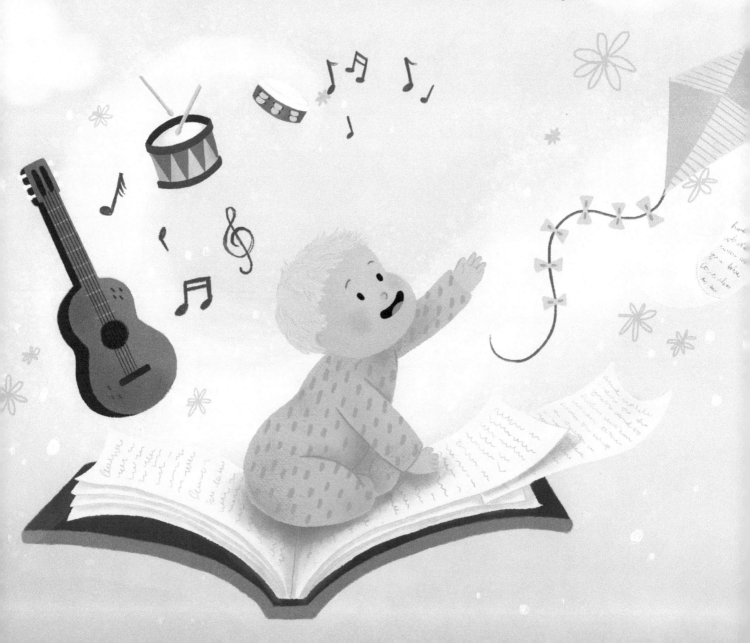

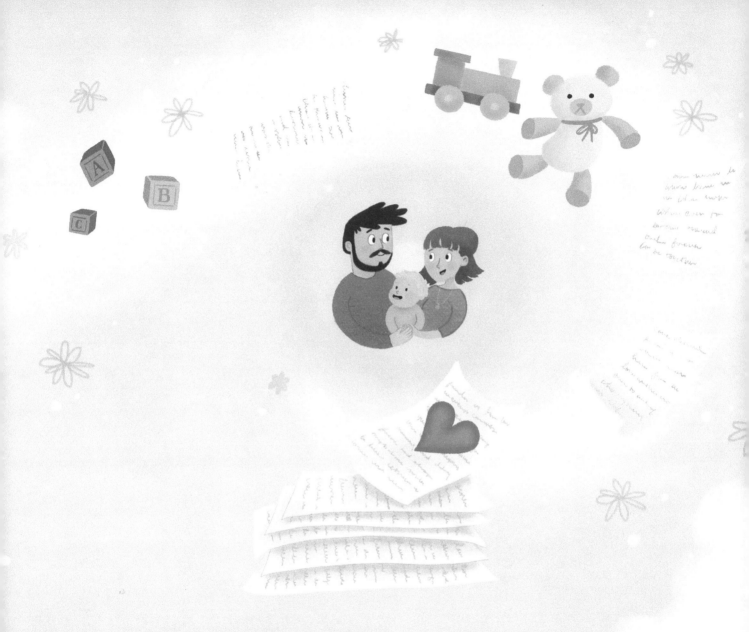

I could never imagine the love that would be,
When I finally knew you were made just for me!

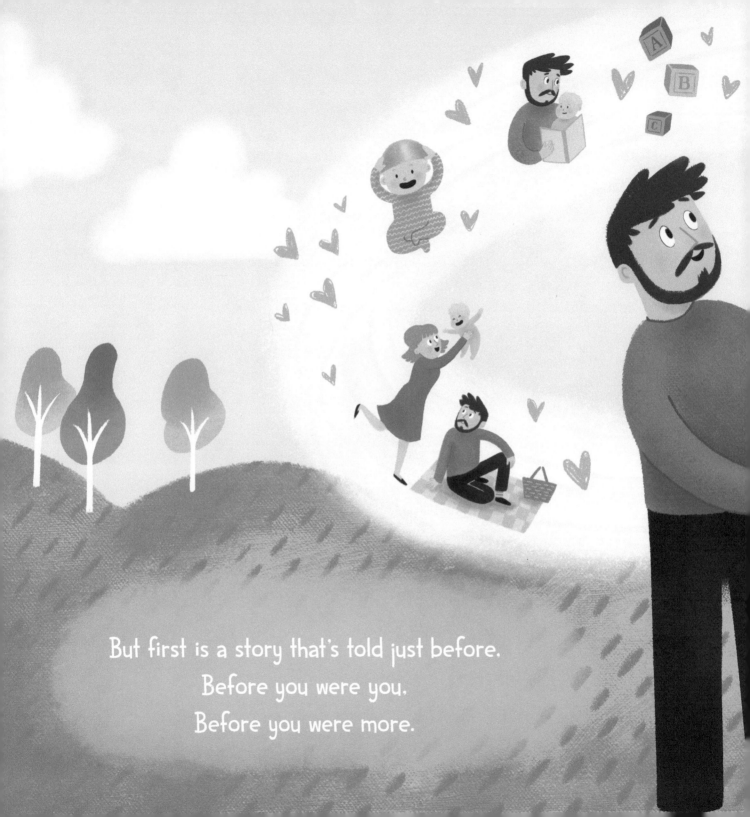

But first is a story that's told just before.
Before you were you.
Before you were more.

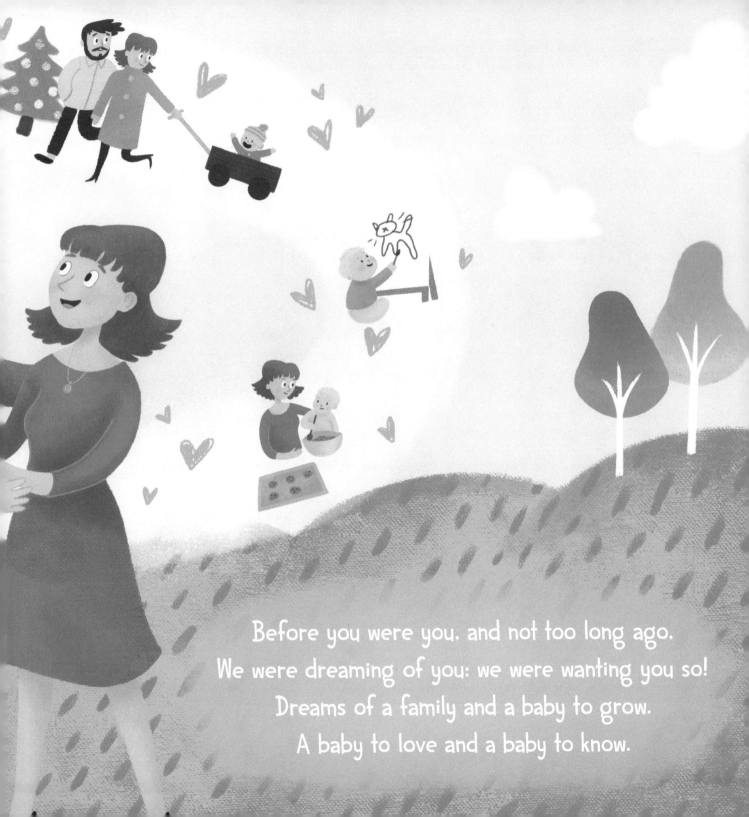

Before you were you. and not too long ago.
We were dreaming of you: we were wanting you so!
Dreams of a family and a baby to grow.
A baby to love and a baby to know.

Just like a puzzle with pieces that fit
To make up a baby, you need quite a bit!
Try as we may and try as we might,
We just couldn't make the pieces fit right.

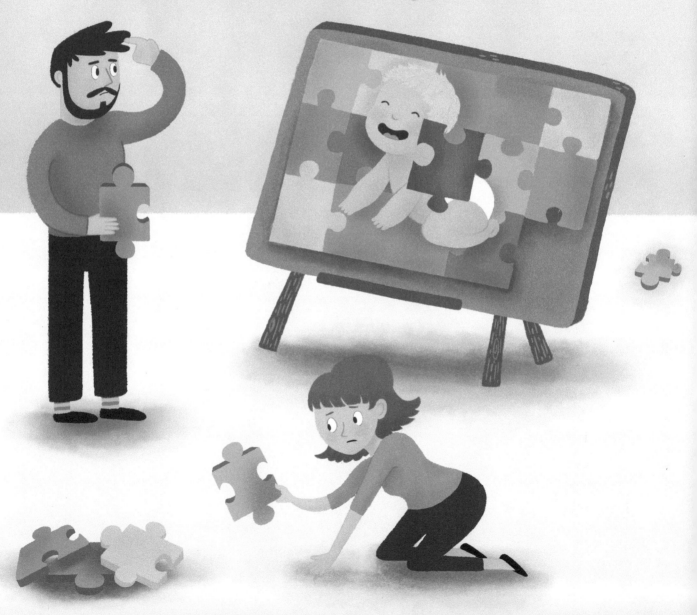

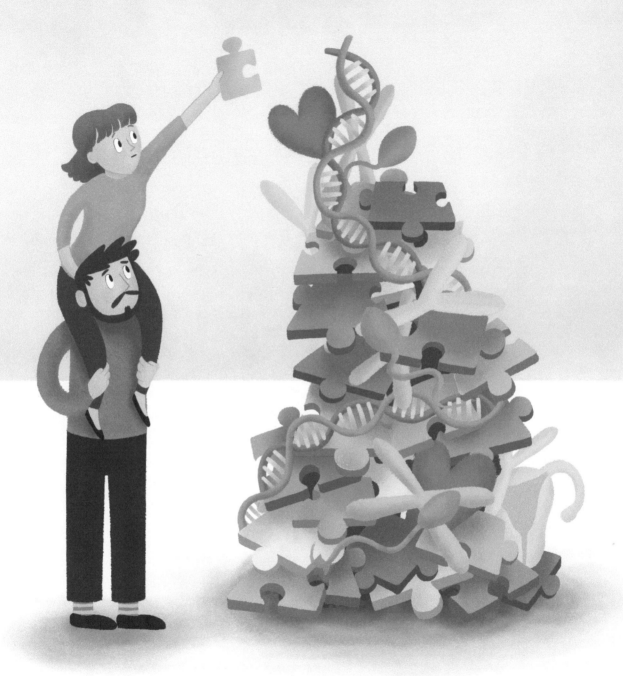

So over and over, we kept trying to try
To fit all the pieces, reaching higher than high.

So out of the house, we finally flew
To ask our wise doctor: *What, oh what, could I do?*

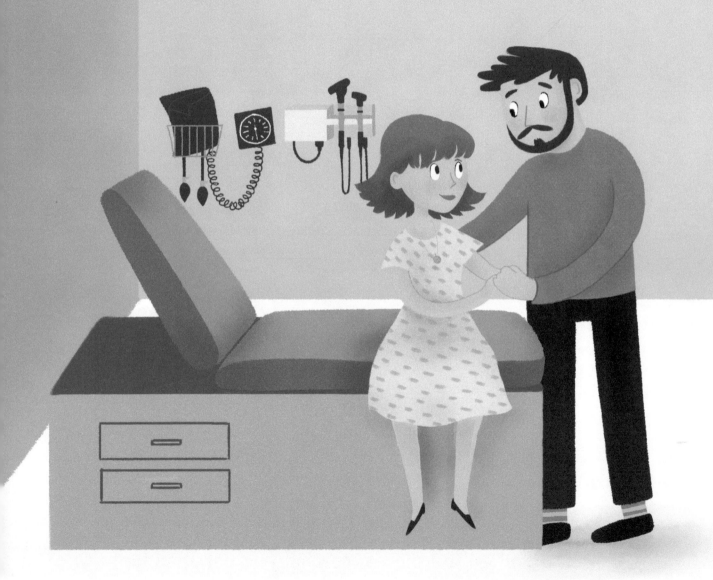

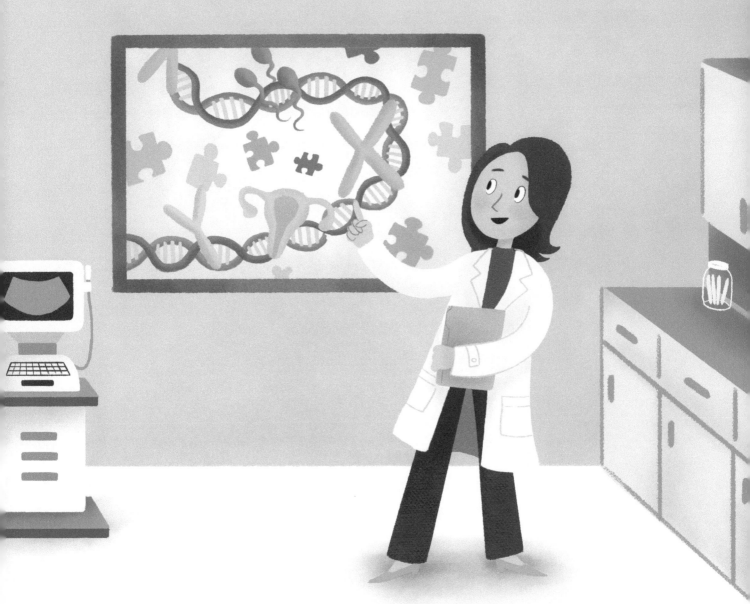

Said the doctor to us, "You have all the pieces just right."
"But you might need some help to make them fit tight."
"I know you are sad," she said with a sigh,
"But there's something amazing, I think we can try."

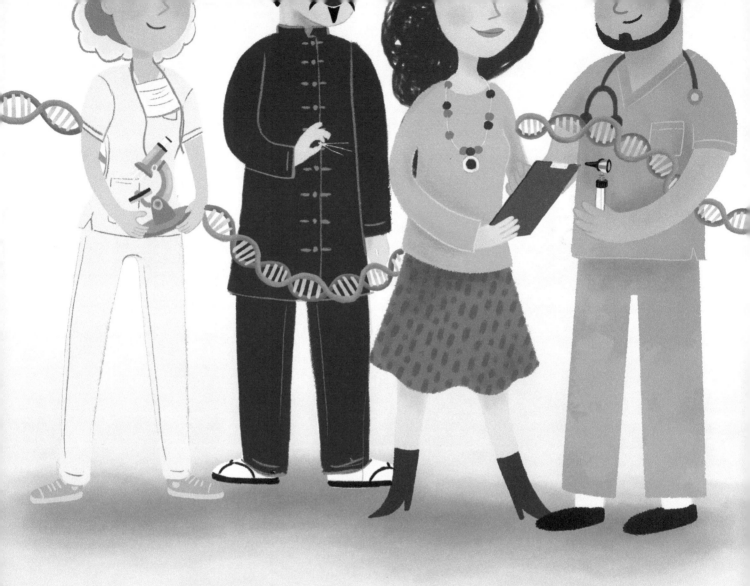

"There are wonderfully helpful people indeed,
Who happen to know how to help you succeed.
With guidance and knowledge they each do their part,
To help grow your family with science and ART."

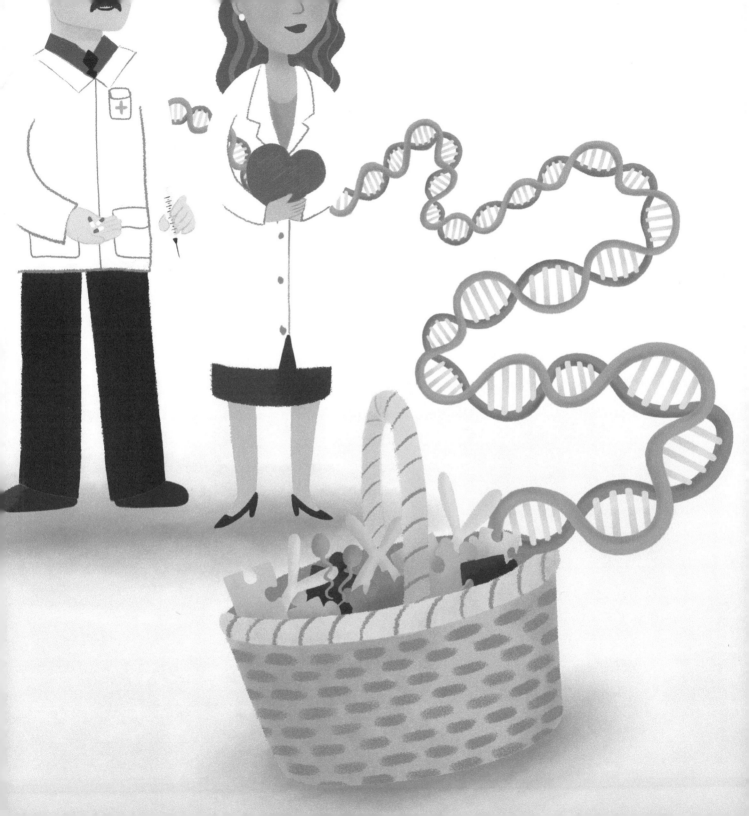

With all of the pieces put together just so,
You went into Mommy's tummy to grow.
From a dot, to a pea, to a melon you grew,
Bigger than big, 'til the day you were due.

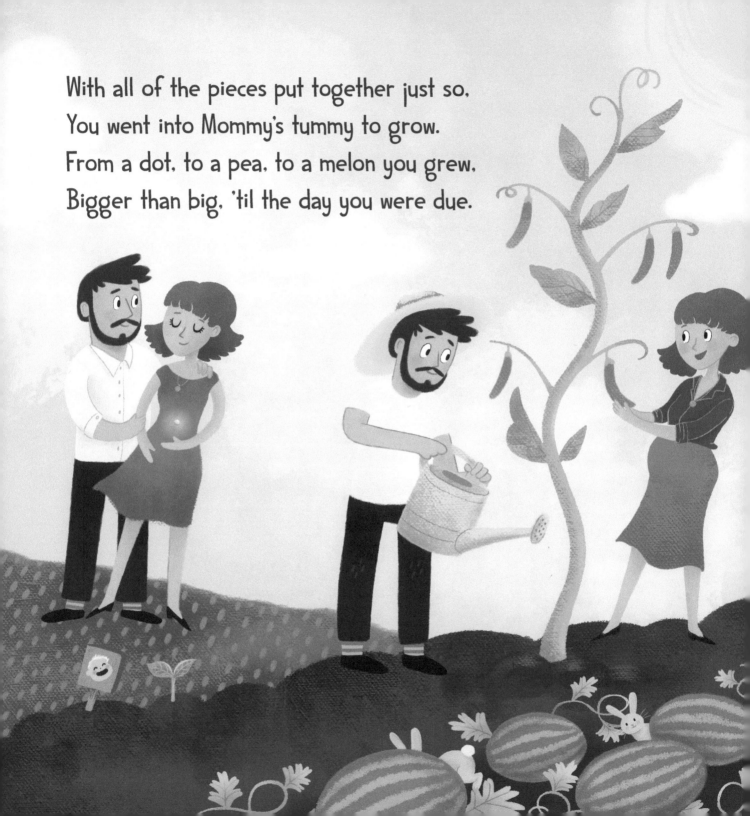

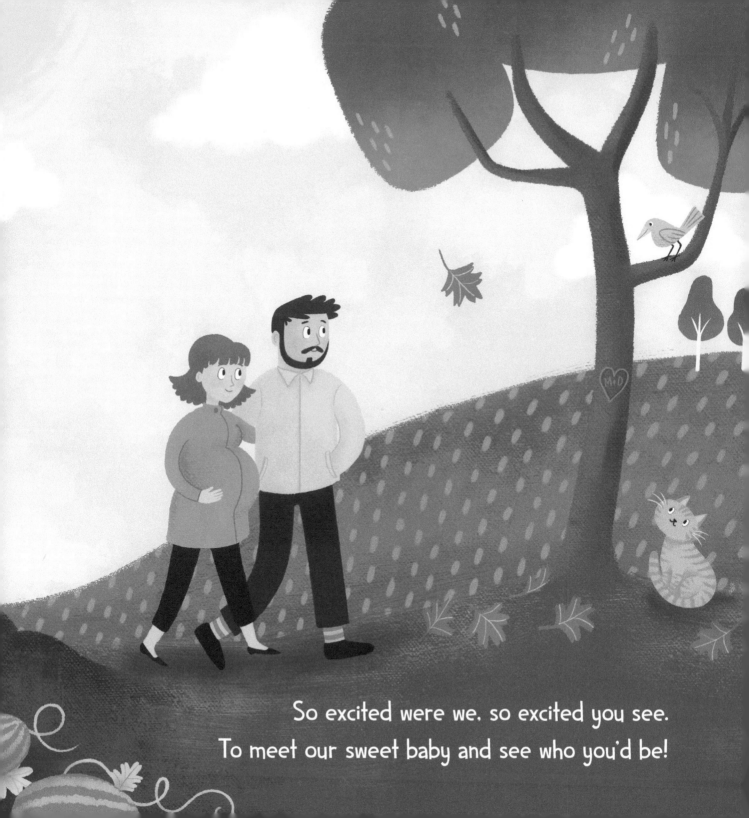

So excited were we, so excited you see.
To meet our sweet baby and see who you'd be!

You entered the world with a cry then a smile,
And snuggled in mommy's warm arms for awhile.
So precious were you: so happy were we:
Everyone shouted with joy, "Yippie!"

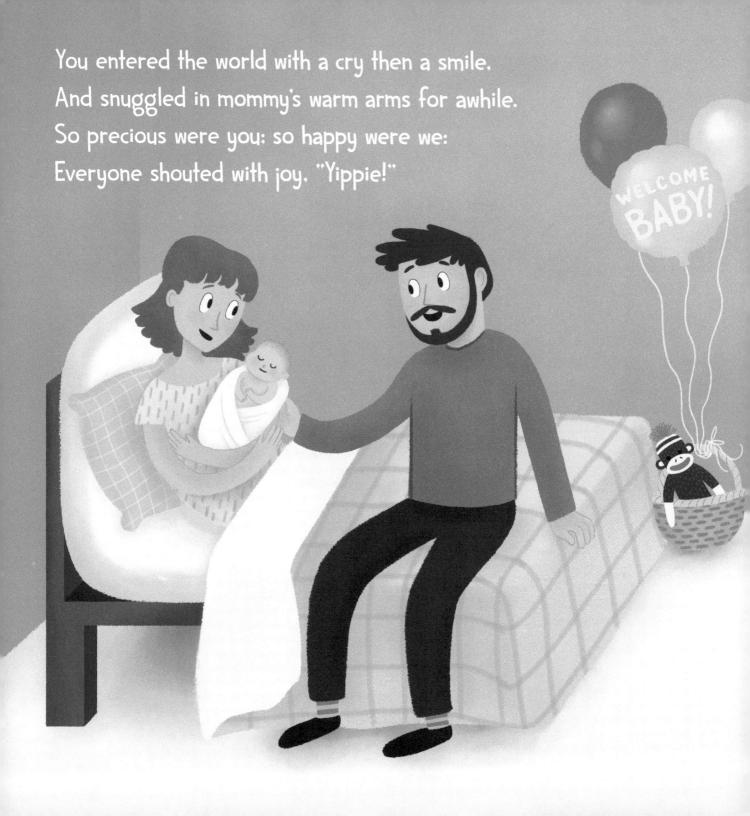

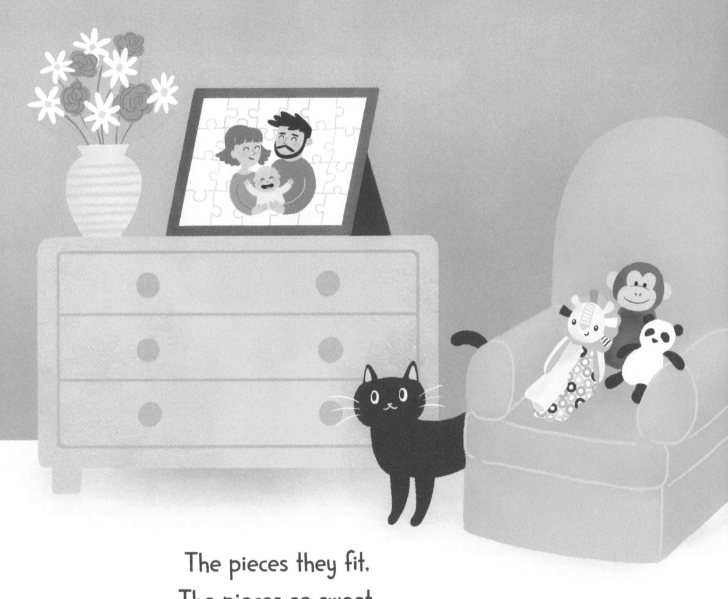

The pieces they fit,
The pieces so sweet.
Our dreams had come true,
The puzzle complete.

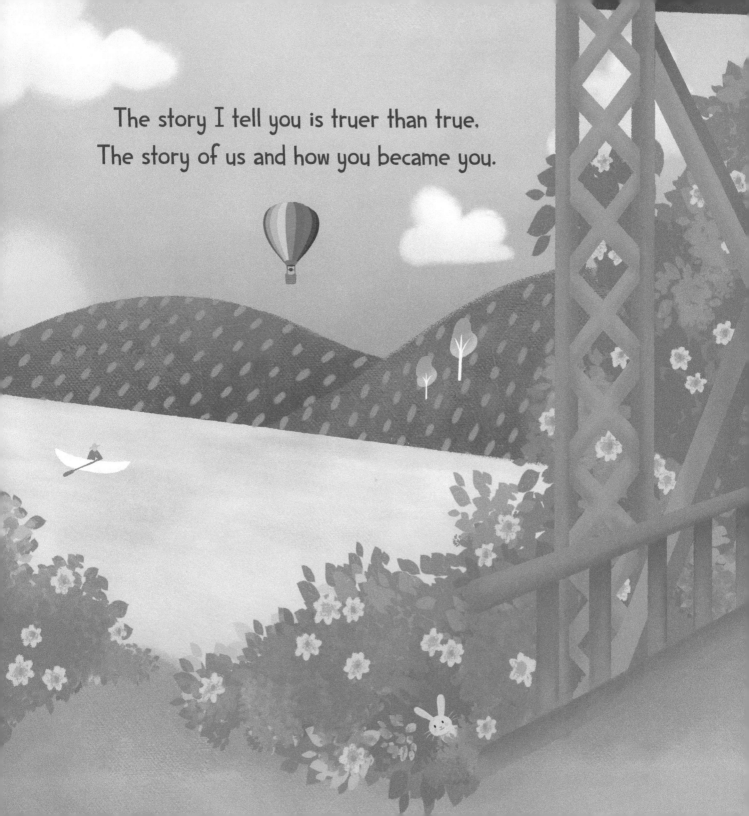

The story I tell you is truer than true,
The story of us and how you became you.

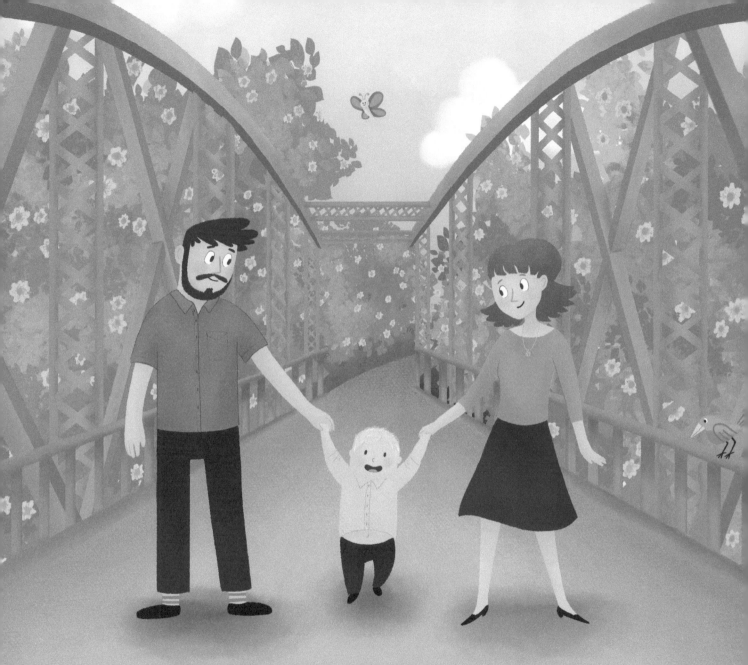

There's no doubt about it you were made just for me,
And forever and ever my baby you'll be!

Questions for your family

Find the heart in the pile of "puzzle pieces". Why do you think this is an important "piece of the puzzle" to make up a baby? What other shapes do you see in the pile? Did your mommy and daddy have all these shapes?

How does the doctor help the mommy in the book make a baby? Did a doctor help your mommy to make you?

What jobs do the "wonderfully helpful people" do for your mommy and daddy so that you could grow?

What things are the "wonderfully helpful people" holding? How do these things help make a baby?

On the day you were born, who was at the hospital to meet you for the first time?

_____

Need help answering these questions?
Visit YouWereMadeForMe.com

WRITE YOUR OWN STORY

Use this page to tell your child's creation story:

_____

_____

_____

_____

_____

_____

_____

_____

_____

_____

CPSIA information can be obtained
at www.ICGtesting.com
Printed in the USA
BVHW012030060220
571677BV00006B/8